ALEXIA M. GREENFIELD

THE ATLANTIC DIET MEAL PLAN

Quick and Easy to Prepare Delicious Recipes for a Healthier You

Contents

1

Introduction

Step into the world of "The Atlantic Diet Meal Plan," where wholesome ingredients, vibrant flavors, and heartwarming stories come together to create a culinary journey like no other. Join us as we explore the rich traditions and coastal delights of the Mediterranean, guided by Sofia, a passionate cook with a deep love for her seaside home.

In this book, you'll discover a treasure trove of simple yet delicious recipes inspired by the bountiful harvests of the Atlantic coast. From succulent seafood dishes to fresh salads bursting with flavor, each recipe is a celebration of the joys of home cooking and the beauty of sharing a meal with loved ones.

So come along and let the pages of "The Atlantic Diet Meal Plan" whisk you away to sun-drenched shores and unforgettable feasts. With every recipe, you'll embark on a culinary adventure that nourishes both body and soul, leaving you feeling satisfied, inspired, and eager to create your own delicious memories.

2

Chapter 1: Understanding the Atlantic Diet

The Atlantic Diet is more than just a collection of foods; it embodies a set of principles and a philosophy that guide its approach to nutrition, health, and well-being. This chapter explores the core principles and underlying philosophy of the Atlantic Diet, providing insight into its holistic approach to food, lifestyle, and sustainability.

1.Emphasis on Fresh, Whole Foods

At the heart of the Atlantic Diet is a focus on fresh, minimally processed foods that are locally sourced and seasonally available. This includes a rich variety of fruits, vegetables, whole grains, legumes, seafood, and lean meats, with an emphasis on quality, flavor, and nutritional density.

By prioritizing whole foods over processed counterparts, the Atlantic Diet aims to maximize nutrient intake while minimizing the consumption of additives, preservatives, and refined ingredients.

2. Diversity and Balance

The Atlantic Diet encourages a diverse and balanced approach to eating, incorporating a wide range of food groups and flavors into meals. By embracing variety, individuals can ensure adequate intake of essential nutrients, antioxidants, and phytochemicals, while also enjoying a more satisfying and culturally rich culinary experience.

Balance is also emphasized in terms of macronutrients, with an emphasis on achieving a healthy ratio of carbohydrates, proteins, and fats. The Atlantic Diet recognizes the importance of each macronutrient for energy, satiety, and metabolic health, while advocating for moderation and mindful eating.

3. Sustainability and Seasonality

Central to the philosophy of the Atlantic Diet is a deep respect for the natural environment and a commitment to sustainable food production practices. This includes supporting local farmers, fishermen, and artisans, minimizing food waste, and preserving biodiversity.

Seasonality plays a crucial role in the Atlantic Diet, with an emphasis on eating foods that are in season and harvested at their peak of freshness. By aligning dietary choices with the rhythm of nature, individuals can reduce their environmental footprint and enjoy the full flavor and nutritional benefits of seasonal produce.

4.Cultural Heritage and Tradition

The Atlantic Diet celebrates the cultural heritage and culinary traditions of the regions surrounding the Atlantic Ocean, paying homage to centuries of gastronomic innovation, craftsmanship, and community rituals. Through food, individuals can connect with their cultural roots, honor ancestral traditions, and foster a sense of belonging and identity.

Traditional cooking methods, recipes, and rituals are preserved and passed down through generations, serving as a source of inspiration and cultural continuity in an increasingly globalized world.

5. Mindful Eating and Pleasure

Mindful eating is a core tenet of the Atlantic Diet, encouraging individuals to cultivate awareness, gratitude, and pleasure in their eating experiences. By savoring each bite, tuning into hunger and satiety cues, and practicing mindful portion control, individuals can develop a healthier relationship with food and enhance their overall well-being.

Pleasure is also considered an essential aspect of the Atlantic Diet, with an emphasis on enjoying food in the company of loved ones, savoring the flavors and textures of seasonal ingredients, and celebrating the joy of shared meals.

Key Components of the Atlantic Diet

1.Fresh Fruits and Vegetables

- Fresh fruits and vegetables are nutrient-dense foods, meaning they provide a high concentration of essential nutrients relative to their calorie content. They are rich sources of vitamins, including vitamin A, vitamin C, vitamin K, and various B vitamins, as well as minerals such as potassium, magnesium, and folate. Each fruit and vegetable offers a unique combination of nutrients, phytochemicals, and antioxidants, contributing to a well-rounded and balanced diet. For example, leafy greens like spinach and kale are rich in vitamin K and folate, while citrus fruits like oranges and grapefruits provide vitamin C and flavonoids.
- Experiment with different cooking methods, seasonings, and flavor combinations to discover new ways to enjoy fresh produce. From simple salads and stir-fries to hearty soups and vegetable-based sauces, there are countless ways to incorporate fruits and vegetables into your meals.

2. Seafood and Fish

- Seafood and fish are excellent sources of high-quality protein, which is essential for muscle repair and growth, immune function, hormone synthesis, and enzyme activity. Unlike many land-based animal protein sources, seafood is typically lower in saturated fat and cholesterol, making it a heart-healthy choice. Consuming adequate protein is particularly important for maintaining muscle mass, supporting weight management, and promoting satiety, helping you feel full and satisfied after meals.

- Incorporate seafood into a variety of dishes, including salads, soups, stews, pasta dishes, tacos, sandwiches, and sushi. From simple grilled fish fillets to elaborate seafood paellas, there are endless ways to enjoy the delicious taste and nutritional benefits of seafood in your meals.

3.Whole Grains and Legumes

- Whole grains and legumes are excellent sources of complex carbohydrates, which provide sustained energy and help regulate blood sugar levels. Unlike refined carbohydrates found in processed grains and sugars, complex carbohydrates are digested more slowly, resulting in a gradual release of glucose into the bloodstream and a more stable energy level.
- Consuming a diet rich in complex carbohydrates can help prevent energy crashes, improve satiety, and support weight management by promoting feelings of fullness and reducing cravings for unhealthy snacks.

4.Healthy Fats

- Healthy fats are an essential component of the Atlantic Diet, providing numerous health benefits and contributing to overall well-being. Unlike saturated and trans fats, which are linked to an increased risk of heart disease and other chronic conditions, healthy fats support cardiovascular health, brain function, hormone production, and inflammation regulation.

Health Benefit of the Atlantic Diet

1. Heart Health: One of the most significant benefits of the Atlantic diet is its positive impact on heart health. It emphasizes the consumption of heart-healthy foods such as fruits, vegetables, whole grains, legumes, nuts, seeds, and olive oil while limiting the intake of red meat and processed foods. These dietary choices are associated with lower rates of cardiovascular disease, including lower blood pressure, reduced risk of heart attack and stroke, and improved cholesterol levels.

2. Reduced Risk of Chronic Diseases: The Atlantic diet has been linked to a lower risk of chronic diseases such as type 2 diabetes, certain cancers (including breast and colorectal cancer), and diseases like Alzheimer's and Parkinson's disease. The abundance of antioxidants, anti-inflammatory compounds, and fiber-rich foods in this diet helps protect against cellular damage and chronic inflammation, which are underlying factors in the development of these diseases.

3. Weight Management: The Atlantic diet emphasizes whole, nutrient-dense foods while minimizing processed and refined foods. This approach naturally leads to a diet that is lower in calories and higher in fiber, which can help with weight management and weight loss. Additionally, the diet's emphasis on healthy fats, lean proteins, and complex carbohydrates promotes satiety, making it easier to maintain a healthy weight over the long term.

4. Improved Cognitive Function: Several studies have suggested that adherence to the Atlantic diet is associated with better cognitive function and a reduced risk of cognitive decline in older adults. The combination of antioxidants, omega-3 fatty acids from seafood, and anti-inflammatory foods in the diet may help protect brain health and preserve cognitive function as we age.

5. Bone Health: The Atlantic diet includes foods rich in calcium, magnesium, vitamin D, and vitamin K, all of which are essential for bone health. Regular consumption of dairy products, leafy greens, nuts, and seafood can help strengthen bones, reduce the risk of osteoporosis, and promote overall bone density and strength.

6. Improved Gut Health: The Atlantic diet is rich in fiber from fruits, vegetables, whole grains, and legumes, which promotes a healthy digestive system and supports beneficial gut bacteria. A healthy gut microbiome is associated with better digestion, nutrient absorption, immune function, and even mental health.

7. Longevity: Studies have consistently shown that populations following a Mediterranean-style diet, including those along the Atlantic coast, tend to have longer life expectancies and lower rates of age-related diseases. The combination of nutritious foods, moderate alcohol consumption (such as red wine), regular physical activity, and a strong sense of community and social connections contribute to overall health and longevity.

3

Chapter 2: Getting Started with the Atlantic Diet

Preparing your Kitchen for the Atlantic Diet

Preparing your kitchen for the Atlantic diet involves setting up an environment that supports your commitment to healthy eating and culinary exploration. Below are some tips on how to get your kitchen ready:

1. Stock Up on Staples

- Extra-Virgin Olive Oil: A staple of the Atlantic diet, extra-virgin olive oil is used for cooking, salad dressings, and drizzling over finished dishes.
- Whole Grains:Keep a variety of whole grains such as brown rice, quinoa, whole wheat pasta, and oats on hand for nutritious meals and snacks.
- Legumes: Stock up on dried or canned legumes like chickpeas, lentils, and beans for protein-rich additions to soups, salads, and stews.
- Canned Tomatoes: Canned tomatoes are versatile ingredients for Mediterranean-inspired sauces, soups, and stews.
- Herbs and Spices: Build a collection of herbs and spices like basil, oregano,

thyme, rosemary, garlic powder, and paprika to add flavor to your dishes without relying on excess salt or sugar.

- Nuts and Seeds: Keep a variety of nuts and seeds such as almonds, walnuts, pumpkin seeds, and chia seeds for snacking and adding crunch to salads and yogurt.
- Seafood: Purchase high-quality frozen or fresh seafood like salmon, tuna, shrimp, and mussels to incorporate into your meals for lean protein and omega-3 fatty acids.
- Fresh Produce: Fill your kitchen with a colorful array of fruits and vegetables, focusing on seasonal options whenever possible. Include staples like tomatoes, cucumbers, bell peppers, spinach, kale, citrus fruits, and berries.

2. Invest in Quality Cookware

- Nonstick Skillet: A nonstick skillet is essential for sautéing vegetables, cooking eggs, and preparing seafood with minimal added oil.
- Chef's Knife and Cutting Board: Invest in a high-quality chef's knife and cutting board for chopping, dicing, and slicing fruits, vegetables, and herbs.
- Baking Sheet and Roasting Pan: Use baking sheets and roasting pans for cooking vegetables, roasting fish, and preparing sheet pan meals.
- Soup Pot and Dutch Oven: These versatile pots are perfect for simmering soups, stews, and sauces, as well as cooking grains and legumes.
- Blender or Food Processor: A blender or food processor is handy for making smoothies, sauces, dips, and homemade salad dressings.

3. Organize Your Pantry

- Arrange your pantry to make healthy choices more accessible. Keep whole grains, legumes, canned tomatoes, and other pantry staples at eye level.
- Use clear containers or labels to identify ingredients and expiration dates

easily.

- Keep healthier options in front and less healthy options hidden or out of reach to encourage better choices.

4. Meal Prep and Batch Cooking

- Dedicate time each week to meal prep and batch cooking. Prepare ingredients in advance, such as washing and chopping vegetables, cooking grains, and marinating proteins, to streamline meal preparation throughout the week.
- Store prepared ingredients in airtight containers or storage bags in the refrigerator or freezer for easy access when cooking.

5. Keep It Clean and Organized

- Maintain a clean and organized kitchen to create an inviting space for cooking and meal preparation.
- Clean stovetops, countertops, and kitchen appliances regularly to prevent cross-contamination and ensure food safety.
- Store kitchen tools and utensils in designated areas for easy access and efficient meal preparation.

shopping for Atlantic diet-Friendly food

Shopping for Atlantic diet-friendly food involves selecting fresh, whole ingredients that are staples of the Mediterranean diet. Below are some tips on how to shop for Atlantic diet-friendly foods:

1. Focus on Fresh Produce

- Start your shopping trip in the produce section. Choose a variety of colorful fruits and vegetables, focusing on seasonal options whenever possible. Opt for leafy greens like spinach and kale, cruciferous vegetables like broccoli and Brussels sprouts, and vibrant bell peppers, tomatoes, cucumbers, and zucchini.
- Select a mix of fresh herbs like basil, parsley, cilantro, and mint to add flavor to your dishes.

2. Choose Lean Proteins

- Look for lean protein sources such as seafood, poultry, and legumes. Choose fresh or frozen fish like salmon, tuna, cod, and shrimp, and consider trying lesser-known varieties like sardines and mackerel, which are rich in omega-3 fatty acids.
- Opt for skinless poultry cuts like chicken breast or turkey breast, and include plant-based protein options such as lentils, chickpeas, and beans.

3. Include Whole Grains and Legumes

- Stock up on whole grains such as brown rice, quinoa, bulgur, farro, and whole wheat pasta. These grains are rich in fiber, vitamins, and minerals and provide a nutritious base for meals.
- Choose a variety of legumes, including canned or dried beans like chickpeas, black beans, kidney beans, and lentils. Legumes are good source of plant-based protein, fiber, and micronutrients.

4. Don't Forget Healthy Fats

- Incorporate heart-healthy fats into your diet by choosing sources like extra-virgin olive oil, avocado, nuts, and seeds. Look for cold-pressed, unrefined olive oil for maximum flavor and nutritional benefits.

- Add nuts and seeds like almonds, walnuts, chia seeds, and flaxseeds to your shopping list for snacking, baking, and adding crunch to salads and yogurt.

5. Explore Dairy and Dairy Alternatives

- Include dairy products like Greek yogurt and feta cheese in your shopping cart for their rich taste and nutritional value. choose low-fat or fat-free options if you're watching your calorie intake.
- Consider dairy alternatives such as unsweetened almond milk, coconut yogurt, and tofu-based cheeses if you're lactose intolerant or following a plant-based diet.

6. Shop the Perimeter of the Store

- When grocery shopping, focus on shopping the perimeter of the store, where you'll find fresh produce, seafood, lean meats, dairy, and whole grains. The interior aisles typically contain processed and packaged foods that may not align with the Atlantic diet.

7. Read Labels Carefully

- When purchasing packaged foods, read labels carefully and choose options with minimal added sugars, sodium, and unhealthy fats. Look for whole food ingredients and avoid products with lengthy ingredient lists and artificial additives.

8. Plan Ahead and Make a List

- Before heading to the grocery store, plan your meals for the week and make a list of ingredients you'll need. This will help you stay organized and avoid impulse purchases of unhealthy items.

4

Chapter 3: Meal Plans and Recipes

Day 1(Week One)

Breakfast: Oatmeal with Fresh Berries

Ingredients

- 1/2 cup rolled oats
- 1 cup water or milk of your choice
- 1/2 cup mixed berries (blueberries, strawberries, raspberries)
- 1 tablespoon chopped nuts (walnuts, almonds)

Instructions

1. In a small saucepan, bring water or milk to a boil.
2. Stir in oats and reduce heat to low. Cook for about 5 minutes, stirring occasionally, until the oats are cooked and the mixture thickens.
3. Transfer the oatmeal to a bowl, top with mixed berries and chopped nuts.

Nutritional Information (approximate per serving)

- Calories: 250
- Protein: 7g
- Carbohydrates: 40g
- Fat: 8g
- Fiber: 6g

Lunch: Grilled Salmon with Steamed Vegetables

Ingredients

- 6 oz salmon fillet
- Assorted vegetables (broccoli, carrots, spinach)
- Olive oil
- Salt and pepper to taste

Instructions

1. Preheat grill to medium-high heat. Brush salmon fillet and vegetables with olive oil, then season with salt and pepper.
2. Grill salmon for about 4-5 minutes on each side, or until cooked through and flaky. Grill vegetables until tender.
3. Serve grilled salmon with steamed vegetables.

Nutritional Information (approximate per serving)
Salmon:

- Calories: 300
- Protein: 34g
- Carbohydrates: 0g
- Fat: 18g
- Fiber: 0g

Vegetables:

- Calories: 50
- Protein: 2g
- Carbohydrates: 10g
- Fat: 1g
- Fiber: 4g

Snack: Greek Yogurt with Honey and Mixed Seeds

Ingredients

- 1/2 cup Greek yogurt
- 1 teaspoon honey
- 1 tablespoon mixed seeds (chia seeds, sunflower seeds)

Instructions

1. In a bowl, mix Greek yogurt with honey.
2. Top with mixed seeds.

Nutritional Information (approximate per serving)

- Calories: 150
- Protein: 15g
- Carbohydrates: 12g
- Fat: 6g
- Fiber: 2g

Dinner: Baked Cod with Roasted Potatoes and Green Beans

Ingredients

- 6 oz cod fillet
- 1 large potato, diced
- 1 cup green beans

- Olive oil
- Salt and pepper to taste

Instructions

1. Preheat oven to 400°F (200°C). Place cod fillet on a baking sheet lined with parchment paper.
2. Toss diced potatoes and green beans with olive oil, salt, and pepper. Spread them around the cod on the baking sheet.
3. Bake for about 15-20 minutes, or until the cod is cooked through and the potatoes are tender.

Nutritional Information (approximate per serving)
Cod:

- Calories: 200
- Protein: 40g
- Carbohydrates: 0g
- Fat: 2g
- Fiber: 0g

Potatoes and Green Beans:

- Calories: 150
- Protein: 4g
- Carbohydrates: 30g
- Fat: 2g
- Fiber: 6g

Day 2

Breakfast: Avocado Toast with Poached Eggs

Ingredients

- 2 slices whole grain bread
- 1 ripe avocado
- 2 eggs
- Salt and pepper to taste

Instructions

1. Toast the whole grain bread slices to your desired level of crispiness.
2. While the bread is toasting, mash the ripe avocado in a bowl and season with salt and pepper.
3. Poach the eggs in simmering water for about 3-4 minutes until the whites are set but the yolks are still runny.
4. Spread the mashed avocado evenly onto the toasted bread slices and top each with a poached egg.

Nutritional Information (approximate per serving)

- Calories: 350
- Protein: 14g
- Carbohydrates: 30g
- Fat: 20g
- Fiber: 10g

Lunch: Grilled Shrimp Skewers with Brown Rice Pilaf

Ingredients

- 6 oz shrimp, peeled and deveined
- Assorted vegetables for skewers (bell peppers, onions)

- 1 cup brown rice
- 1/2 cup peas
- 1/2 cup diced carrots
- Olive oil
- Salt and pepper to taste

Instructions

1. Preheat grill to medium-high heat. Thread assorted vegetables and shrimp onto skewers.
2. Grill shrimp skewers for about 2-3 minutes on each side until shrimp are pink and opaque.
3. Cook brown rice according to package instructions. In a separate pan, sauté peas and carrots with olive oil until tender.
4. Serve grilled shrimp skewers with brown rice pilaf.

Nutritional Information (approximate per serving)
Shrimp Skewers:

- Calories: 200
- Protein: 24g
- Carbohydrates: 6g
- Fat: 8g
- Fiber: 1g

Brown Rice Pilaf:

- Calories: 250
- Protein: 5g
- Carbohydrates: 50g
- Fat: 2g
- Fiber: 5g

Snack: Apple Slices with Almond Butter

Ingredients

- 1 apple, sliced
- 2 tablespoons almond butter

Instructions

1. Slice the apple into wedges.
2. Dip apple slices into almond butter before each bite.

Nutritional Information (approximate per serving)

- Calories: 200
- Protein: 4g
- Carbohydrates: 20g
- Fat: 14g
- Fiber: 6g

Dinner: Baked Haddock with Quinoa and Black Bean Salad

Ingredients

- 6 oz haddock fillet
- 1 cup quinoa, cooked
- 1/2 cup black beans, drained and rinsed
- Assorted diced vegetables (bell peppers, corn)
- Fresh cilantro, chopped
- Lime juice
- Olive oil
- Salt and pepper to taste

Instructions

1. Preheat oven to 375°F (190°C). Place haddock fillet on a baking sheet lined with parchment paper.
2. Drizzle haddock with olive oil and lime juice, then season with salt and pepper. Bake for about 15-20 minutes until fish flakes easily with a fork.
3. In a bowl, combine cooked quinoa, black beans, diced vegetables, chopped cilantro, olive oil, and lime juice. Season with salt and pepper to taste.
4. Serve baked haddock with quinoa and black bean salad.

Nutritional Information (approximate per serving)
Haddock:

- Calories: 200
- Protein: 30g
- Carbohydrates: 0g
- Fat: 8g
- Fiber: 0g

Quinoa and Black Bean Salad:

- Calories: 300
- Protein: 10g
- Carbohydrates: 45g
- Fat: 8g
- Fiber: 10g

Day 3

Breakfast: Blueberry Greek Yogurt Parfait

Ingredients

- 1 cup Greek yogurt

- 1/2 cup fresh blueberries
- 1/4 cup granola
- 1 tablespoon honey (optional)

Instructions

1. In a glass or bowl, layer Greek yogurt, fresh blueberries, and granola.
2. Drizzle with honey if desired.

Nutritional Information (approximate per serving)

- Calories: 250
- Protein: 18g
- Carbohydrates: 35g
- Fat: 6g
- Fiber: 4g

Lunch: Tuna Salad Wrap

Ingredients

- 1 can tuna, drained
- 2 tablespoons Greek yogurt
- 1 tablespoon lemon juice
- 1/4 cup diced celery
- 1/4 cup diced red onion
- 2 large lettuce leaves
- 2 whole grain wraps

Instructions

1. In a bowl, mix together tuna, Greek yogurt, lemon juice, diced celery, and diced red onion.

2. Place a lettuce leaf on each wrap, then spoon tuna salad onto the lettuce leaves.

3. Roll up the wraps and slice in half.

Nutritional Information (approximate per serving)

- Calories: 300
- Protein: 30g
- Carbohydrates: 30g
- Fat: 8g
- Fiber: 6g

Snack: Carrot Sticks with Hummus

Ingredients

- 2 medium carrots, peeled and sliced into sticks
- 1/4 cup hummus

Instructions

1. Serve carrot sticks with hummus for dipping.

Nutritional Information (approximate per serving)

- Calories: 100
- Protein: 3g
- Carbohydrates: 15g
- Fat: 4g
- Fiber: 5g

Dinner: Grilled Chicken with Roasted Vegetables

Ingredients

- 6 oz chicken breast
- Assorted vegetables (zucchini, bell peppers, cherry tomatoes)
- Olive oil
- Garlic powder
- Italian seasoning
- Salt and pepper to taste

Instructions

1. Preheat grill to medium-high heat. Season chicken breast with garlic powder, Italian seasoning, salt, and pepper.
2. Grill chicken for about 6-7 minutes on each side until cooked through.
3. Toss assorted vegetables with olive oil, pepper and salt. Spread them on a baking sheet and roast in the oven at 400°F (200°C) for about 15-20 minutes until tender.
4. Serve grilled chicken with roasted vegetables.

Nutritional Information (approximate per serving)
Grilled Chicken:

- Calories: 250
- Protein: 40g
- Carbohydrates: 0g
- Fat: 8g
- Fiber: 0g

Roasted Vegetables:

- Calories: 150

- Protein: 4g
- Carbohydrates: 15g
- Fat: 6g
- Fiber: 6g

Day 4

Breakfast: Smoked Salmon and Avocado Toast

Ingredients

- 2 slices whole grain bread
- 1/2 ripe avocado
- 2 oz smoked salmon
- Lemon juice
- Salt and pepper to taste

Instructions

1. Toast the whole grain bread slices.
2. Mash the ripe avocado and spread it evenly onto the toasted bread slices.
3. Top each toast with smoked salmon slices.
4. Squeeze lemon juice all over the salmon and season with pepper and salt.

Nutritional Information (approximate per serving)

- Calories: 300
- Protein: 20g
- Carbohydrates: 20g
- Fat: 15g
- Fiber: 6g

Lunch: Mediterranean Chickpea Salad

Ingredients

- 1 can chickpeas, drained and rinsed
- 1 cucumber, diced
- 1 tomato, diced
- 1/4 cup diced red onion
- 1/4 cup chopped fresh parsley
- 2 tablespoons olive oil
- 1 tablespoon lemon juice
- Salt and pepper to taste

Instructions

1. In a large bowl, combine chickpeas, diced cucumber, diced tomato, diced red onion, and chopped parsley.
2. Drizzle olive oil and lemon juice over the salad, then toss to coat evenly.
3. Season with salt and pepper to taste.

Nutritional Information (approximate per serving)

- Calories: 250
- Protein: 8g
- Carbohydrates: 30g
- Fat: 10g
- Fiber: 10g

Snack: Mixed Nuts and Dried Fruits

Ingredients

- 1/4 cup mixed nuts (almonds, cashews, walnuts)

- 1/4 cup mixed dried fruits (raisins, apricots, cranberries)

Instructions:

1. Mix the nuts and dried fruits together in a bowl.
2. Portion out the desired amount for a snack.

Nutritional Information (approximate per serving)

- Calories: 200
- Protein: 5g
- Carbohydrates: 20g
- Fat: 12g
- Fiber: 4g

Dinner: Grilled Swordfish with Quinoa Salad

Ingredients

- 6 oz swordfish steak
- 1 cup cooked quinoa
- 1/2 cup cherry tomatoes, halved
- 1/4 cup diced cucumber
- 1/4 cup diced red onion
- 1/4 cup crumbled feta cheese
- Fresh mint leaves, chopped
- Lemon vinaigrette dressing

Instructions

1. Preheat grill to medium-high heat. Season swordfish steak with salt and pepper.
2. Grill swordfish for about 4-5 minutes on each side until cooked through.
3. In a large bowl, combine cooked quinoa, halved cherry tomatoes, diced cucumber, diced red onion, crumbled feta cheese, and chopped mint

leaves.

4. Drizzle lemon vinaigrette dressing over the quinoa salad and toss to combine.
5. Serve grilled swordfish with quinoa salad.

Nutritional Information (approximate per serving)
Grilled Swordfish:

- Calories: 250
- Protein: 40g
- Carbohydrates: 0g
- Fat: 8g
- Fiber: 0g

Quinoa Salad:

- Calories: 300
- Protein: 10g
- Carbohydrates: 40g
- Fat: 10g
- Fiber: 6g

Day 5

Breakfast: Berry Smoothie Bowl

Ingredients

- 1 cup mixed berries (strawberries, blueberries, raspberries)
- 1/2 banana, frozen
- 1/2 cup Greek yogurt
- 1/4 cup any milk of your choice
- Toppings: sliced fresh fruit, granola, chia seeds, shredded coconut

Instructions

1. In a blender, combine mixed berries, frozen banana, Greek yogurt, and almond milk. Blend until smooth.
2. Pour the smoothie into a bowl.
3. Top with sliced fresh fruit, granola, chia seeds, and shredded coconut.

Nutritional Information (approximate per serving)

- Calories: 250
- Protein: 10g
- Carbohydrates: 40g
- Fat: 6g
- Fiber: 8g

Lunch: Grilled Vegetable and Feta Cheese Salad

Ingredients

- Assorted vegetables (bell peppers, zucchini, eggplant), sliced
- Olive oil
- Salt and pepper to taste
- Mixed salad greens
- Crumbled feta cheese
- Balsamic vinaigrette dressing

Instructions

1. Preheat grill to medium-high heat. Toss sliced vegetables with olive oil, salt, and pepper.
2. Grill vegetables for about 3-4 minutes on each side until tender and grill marks appear.
3. Arrange mixed salad greens on a plate. Top it with crumbled feta cheese

and grilled vegetables.

4. Drizzle balsamic vinaigrette dressing over the salad.

Nutritional Information (approximate per serving)

- Calories: 200
- Protein: 8g
- Carbohydrates: 15g
- Fat: 12g
- Fiber: 6g

Snack: Greek Yogurt with Berries and Honey

Ingredients

- 1/2 cup Greek yogurt
- 1/4 cup mixed berries (strawberries, blueberries, raspberries)
- 1 teaspoon honey

Instructions

1. In a bowl, mix Greek yogurt with mixed berries.
2. Drizzle honey over the top.

Nutritional Information (approximate per serving)

- Calories: 150
- Protein: 10g
- Carbohydrates: 20g
- Fat: 2g
- Fiber: 4g

Dinner: Baked Salmon with Lemon Herb Sauce

Ingredients

- 6 oz salmon fillet
- 1 tablespoon olive oil
- 1 tablespoon lemon juice
- 1 teaspoon Dijon mustard
- 1 garlic clove, minced
- 1 tablespoon fresh herbs (such as dill, parsley, or thyme), chopped
- Salt and pepper to taste

Instructions

1. Preheat oven to 375°F (190°C). Place salmon fillet on a baking sheet lined with parchment paper.
2. In a small bowl, whisk together olive oil, lemon juice, Dijon mustard, minced garlic, chopped herbs, salt, and pepper.
3. Pour the lemon herb sauce over the salmon fillet.
4. Bake for about 15-20 minutes until the salmon is cooked through and flakes easily with a fork.

Nutritional Information (approximate per serving)

- Calories: 300
- Protein: 30g
- Carbohydrates: 2g
- Fat: 18g
- Fiber: 0g

Day 6

Breakfast: Spinach and Feta Omelette

Ingredients

- 2 large eggs
- Handful of spinach leaves
- 2 tablespoons crumbled feta cheese
- Salt and pepper to taste

Instructions

1. Beat the eggs In a bowl and season with salt and pepper.
2. Heat a non-stick skillet over medium heat and add the beaten eggs.
3. Once the eggs start to set, add the spinach leaves and crumbled feta cheese on one side of the omelette.
4. Fold the other side of the omelette over the filling and cook for another minute until the cheese melts and the omelette is cooked through.

Nutritional Information (approximate per serving)

- Calories: 250
- Protein: 18g
- Carbohydrates: 3g
- Fat: 18g
- Fiber: 1g

Lunch: Grilled Vegetable Panini

Ingredients

- Assorted vegetables (zucchini, bell peppers, onions, mushrooms), sliced
- Whole grain bread
- Olive oil

- Balsamic vinegar
- Salt and pepper to taste
- Optional: sliced mozzarella cheese

Instructions

1. Preheat grill or grill pan over medium-high heat. Toss the sliced vegetables with olive oil, balsamic vinegar, salt, and pepper.
2. Grill the vegetables for about 3-4 minutes on each side until tender.
3. Assemble the panini by layering the grilled vegetables (and mozzarella cheese if using) between slices of whole grain bread.
4. Grill the assembled panini in a panini press or skillet until the bread is toasted and the cheese is melted.

Nutritional Information (approximate per serving)

- Calories: 300 (without cheese)
- Protein: 8g
- Carbohydrates: 45g
- Fat: 10g
- Fiber: 8g

Snack: Sliced Cucumber with Hummus

Ingredients

- 1 cucumber, sliced
- 1/4 cup hummus

Instructions

1. Serve cucumber slices with hummus for dipping.
Nutritional Information (approximate per serving)

- Calories: 100
- Protein: 4g
- Carbohydrates: 15g
- Fat: 4g
- Fiber: 6g

Dinner: Shrimp and Vegetable Stir-Fry

Ingredients

- 6 oz shrimp, peeled and deveined
- Assorted vegetables (bell peppers, broccoli, carrots, snap peas), sliced
- 2 tablespoons soy sauce
- 1 tablespoon sesame oil
- 1 garlic clove, minced
- 1 teaspoon grated ginger
- Cooked brown rice

Instructions

1. Heat sesame oil in a large skillet over medium-high heat. Add grated ginger and minced garlic and stir-fry for about 30 seconds.
2. Add the sliced vegetables to the skillet and stir-fry for 3-4 minutes until they start to soften.
3. Push the vegetables to the side of the skillet and add the shrimp. Cook until the shrimp turn pink and opaque.
4. Stir in soy sauce and toss everything together until well combined.
5. Serve the shrimp and vegetable stir-fry over cooked brown rice.

Nutritional Information (approximate per serving)

- Calories: 350
- Protein: 30g

- Carbohydrates: 40g
- Fat: 8g
- Fiber: 6g

Day 7

Breakfast: Mediterranean Breakfast Bowl

Ingredients

- 1/2 cup cooked quinoa
- 1/4 cup cherry tomatoes, halved
- 1/4 cup diced cucumber
- 2 tablespoons crumbled feta cheese
- 2 tablespoons Kalamata olives, sliced
- 1 tablespoon chopped fresh parsley
- 1 tablespoon extra virgin olive oil
- Salt and pepper to taste

Instructions

1. In a bowl, combine cooked quinoa, cherry tomatoes, diced cucumber, crumbled feta cheese, sliced Kalamata olives, and chopped fresh parsley.
2. Drizzle extra virgin olive oil over the bowl and season with salt and pepper.

Nutritional Information (approximate per serving)

- Calories: 300
- Protein: 8g
- Carbohydrates: 20g
- Fat: 18g
- Fiber: 4g

Lunch: Tuna Stuffed Bell Peppers

Ingredients

- 2 large bell peppers, halved and seeded
- 1 can tuna, drained
- 1/4 cup diced red onion
- 1/4 cup diced cucumber
- 1/4 cup diced tomato
- 2 tablespoons Greek yogurt
- 1 tablespoon lemon juice
- Salt and pepper to taste

Instructions

1. Preheat oven to 375°F (190°C). Place bell pepper halves in a baking dish.
2. In a bowl, mix together drained tuna, diced red onion, diced cucumber, diced tomato, Greek yogurt, lemon juice, salt, and pepper.
3. Spoon the tuna mixture into each bell pepper half.
4. Bake for about 20-25 minutes until the bell peppers are tender.

Nutritional Information (approximate per serving)

- Calories: 250
- Protein: 30g
- Carbohydrates: 15g
- Fat: 8g
- Fiber: 4g

Snack: Apple Slices with Almond Butter

Ingredients

- 1 apple, sliced
- 2 tablespoons almond butter

Instructions

1. Slice the apple into wedges.
2. Dip apple slices into almond butter before each bite.

Nutritional Information (approximate per serving)

- Calories: 200
- Protein: 4g
- Carbohydrates: 20g
- Fat: 14g
- Fiber: 6g

Dinner: Grilled Swordfish with Mango Salsa

Ingredients

- 6 oz swordfish steak
- 1 ripe mango, diced
- 1/4 cup diced red onion
- 1/4 cup chopped fresh cilantro
- 1 jalapeno pepper, seeded and minced
- Juice of 1 lime
- Salt and pepper to taste

Instructions

1. Preheat grill to medium-high heat. Season swordfish steak with salt and

pepper.

2. Grill swordfish for about 4-5 minutes on each side until cooked through.
3. In a bowl, mix together diced mango, diced red onion, chopped cilantro, minced jalapeno pepper, lime juice, salt, and pepper to make the salsa.
4. Serve grilled swordfish topped with mango salsa.

Nutritional Information (approximate per serving)

- Calories: 300
- Protein: 30g
- Carbohydrates: 20g
- Fat: 8g
- Fiber: 4g

Day 1(Week 2)

Breakfast: Banana Walnut Overnight Oats

Ingredients

- 1/2 cup rolled oats
- 1/2 cup any milk of your choice
- 1/2 ripe banana, mashed
- 1 tablespoon chopped walnuts
- 1 tablespoon honey (optional)

Instructions

1. In a jar or bowl, mix together rolled oats and almond milk.
2. Stir in mashed banana and chopped walnuts.
3. Cover and refrigerate overnight.

4. In the morning, drizzle with honey if desired before serving.

Nutritional Information (approximate per serving)

- Calories: 300
- Protein: 7g
- Carbohydrates: 45g
- Fat: 10g
- Fiber: 6g

Lunch: Greek Salad with Grilled Chicken

Ingredients

- Mixed salad greens
- 4 oz grilled chicken breast, sliced
- 1/4 cup cherry tomatoes, halved
- 1/4 cup sliced cucumber
- 2 tablespoons sliced red onion
- 2 tablespoons Kalamata olives
- 2 tablespoons crumbled feta cheese
- Greek vinaigrette dressing

Instructions

1. Arrange mixed salad greens on a plate.
2. Top with sliced grilled chicken breast, cherry tomatoes, sliced cucumber, sliced red onion, Kalamata olives, and crumbled feta cheese.
3. Drizzle with Greek vinaigrette dressing.

Nutritional Information (approximate per serving)

- Calories: 350

- Protein: 30g
- Carbohydrates: 15g
- Fat: 18g
- Fiber: 4g

Snack: Hummus with Whole Grain Crackers

Ingredients

- 1/4 cup hummus
- Whole grain crackers

Instructions

1. Serve hummus with whole grain crackers for dipping.
Nutritional Information (approximate per serving)

- Calories: 150
- Protein: 5g
- Carbohydrates: 20g
- Fat: 6g
- Fiber: 4g

Dinner: Baked Cod with Tomato Basil Sauce

Ingredients

- 6 oz cod fillet
- 1 cup cherry tomatoes
- 1 garlic clove, minced
- 1/4 cup chopped fresh basil
- 1 tablespoon olive oil
- Salt and pepper to taste

Instructions

1. Preheat oven to 375°F (190°C). Place cod fillet on a baking sheet lined with parchment paper.
2. In a bowl, mix together cherry tomatoes, minced garlic, chopped fresh basil, olive oil, salt, and pepper.
3. Spoon the tomato basil mixture over the cod fillet.
4. Bake for about 15-20 minutes until the cod is cooked through and flakes easily with a fork.

Nutritional Information (approximate per serving)

- Calories: 250
- Protein: 30g
- Carbohydrates: 10g
- Fat: 10g

Day 2:

Breakfast: Blueberry Spinach Smoothie

Ingredients

- 1 cup spinach leaves
- 1/2 cup blueberries
- 1/2 banana
- 1/2 cup Greek yogurt
- 1/2 cup any milk of your choice)
- 1 tablespoon honey (optional)

Instructions

1. Combine spinach leaves, blueberries, banana, Greek yogurt, and almond

milk in a blender.
2. Blend until smooth.
3. Taste and add honey if desired.

Nutritional Information (approximate per serving)

- Calories: 200
- Protein: 10g
- Carbohydrates: 35g
- Fat: 3g
- Fiber: 6g

Lunch: Quinoa Salad with Roasted Vegetables

Ingredients

- 1 cup cooked quinoa
- Assorted roasted vegetables (such as bell peppers, zucchini, carrots)
- tablespoons crumbled feta cheese
- 2 tablespoons balsamic vinaigrette dressing

Instructions
1. In a bowl, combine cooked quinoa and roasted vegetables.
2. Top with crumbled feta cheese and balsamic vinaigrette dressing.
3. Toss gently to combine.

Nutritional Information (approximate per serving)

- Calories: 300
- Protein: 8g
- Carbohydrates: 40g
- Fat: 10g
- Fiber: 8g

Snack: Sliced Bell Peppers with Guacamole

Ingredients

- 1 bell pepper, sliced
- 1/2 avocado
- 1/4 onion, finely chopped
- 1/4 tomato, diced
- 1/2 lime, juiced
- Salt and pepper to taste

Instructions

1. In a bowl, mash the avocado with a fork.
2. Add chopped onion, diced tomato, lime juice, salt, and pepper to the mashed avocado, and mix well to make guacamole.
3. Serve sliced bell peppers with guacamole for dipping.

Nutritional Information (approximate per serving)

- Calories: 150
- Protein: 3g
- Carbohydrates: 10g
- Fat: 12g
- Fiber: 5g

Dinner: Lemon Garlic Shrimp Pasta

Ingredients

- 6 oz whole wheat pasta
- 6 oz shrimp, peeled and deveined
- 2 tablespoons olive oil

- 2 cloves garlic, minced
- Zest and juice of 1 lemon
- Salt and pepper to taste
- Fresh parsley, chopped (for garnish)

Instructions

1. Cook pasta according to package instructions. Drain and set aside.
2. In a skillet, heat olive oil over medium heat. Add minced garlic and cook until fragrant.
3. Add shrimp to the skillet and cook until pink and opaque.
4. Stir in lemon zest and juice. Season with salt and pepper.
5. Add cooked pasta to the skillet and toss to coat with the lemon garlic sauce.
6. Serve hot, garnished with chopped fresh parsley.

Nutritional Information (approximate per serving)

- Calories: 400
- Protein: 25g
- Carbohydrates: 45g
- Fat: 15g
- Fiber: 8g

Day 3

Breakfast: Mediterranean Frittata

Ingredients

- 4 large eggs
- 1/4 cup diced tomatoes
- 1/4 cup chopped spinach

- 2 tablespoons diced red onion
- 2 tablespoons crumbled feta cheese
- Salt and pepper to taste

Instructions

1. Preheat oven to 350°F (175°C).
2. In a bowl, whisk together the eggs, diced tomatoes, chopped spinach, diced red onion, crumbled feta cheese, salt, and pepper.
3. Pour the egg mixture into a greased oven safe skillet.
4. Bake in the preheated oven for 15-20 minutes until the frittata is set and golden brown on top.
5. Slice and serve.

Nutritional Information (approximate per serving)

- Calories: 250
- Protein: 18g
- Carbohydrates: 5g
- Fat: 18g
- Fiber: 2g

Lunch: Caprese Salad

Ingredients

- 1 large tomato, sliced
- 4 oz fresh mozzarella cheese, sliced
- Fresh basil leaves
- 1 tablespoon balsamic glaze
- Salt and pepper to taste

Instructions

1. Arrange alternating slices of tomato and mozzarella cheese on a serving plate.
2. put fresh basil leaves in between the tomato and mozzarella slices.
3. sprinkle with balsamic glaze and season with pepper and salt.

Nutritional Information (approximate per serving)

- Calories: 300
- Protein: 20g
- Carbohydrates: 5g
- Fat: 22g
- Fiber: 1g

Snack: Greek Yogurt with Honey and Walnuts

Ingredients

- 1/2 cup Greek yogurt
- 1 tablespoon honey
- 2 tablespoons chopped walnuts

Instructions

1. In a bowl, combine Greek yogurt and honey.
2. Top with chopped walnuts.

Nutritional Information (approximate per serving)

- Calories: 200
- Protein: 15g
- Carbohydrates: 15g
- Fat: 10g
- Fiber: 1g

Dinner: Lemon Herb Grilled Chicken

Ingredients

- 6 oz chicken breast
- 1 tablespoon olive oil
- Zest and juice of 1 lemon
- 1 clove garlic, minced
- 1 tablespoon chopped fresh herbs (such as oregano, rosemary or thyme)
- Salt and pepper to taste

Instructions

1. In a bowl, whisk together olive oil, lemon zest, lemon juice, minced garlic, chopped fresh herbs, salt, and pepper.
2. Place chicken breast in a resealable plastic bag. Pour the marinade over the chicken, ensuring it is well coated. Marinate in the refrigerator for at least 30 minutes.
3. Preheat grill to medium-high heat. Remove chicken from marinade and discard the excess marinade.
4. Grill chicken for about 6-7 minutes on each side until cooked through and juices run clear.
5. Serve hot.

Nutritional Information (approximate per serving)

- Calories: 300
- Protein: 40g
- Carbohydrates: 2g
- Fat: 14g
- Fiber: 0g

Day 4

Breakfast: Berry Chia Seed Pudding

Ingredients

- 1/4 cup chia seeds
- 1 cup any milk of your choice)
- 1/2 cup mixed berries (strawberries, blueberries, raspberries)
- 1 tablespoon honey (optional)

Instructions

1. In a bowl or jar, mix together chia seeds and almond milk. Stir well to combine.
2. Leave the mixture sit for about 5 minutes, then stir again to prevent clumping.
3. Cover and refrigerate overnight, or for at least 2 hours, until the chia seeds have absorbed the liquid and the mixture has thickened to a pudding-like consistency.
4. Before serving, top with mixed berries and drizzle with honey if desired.

Nutritional Information (approximate per serving)

- Calories: 250
- Protein: 6g
- Carbohydrates: 35g
- Fat: 10g
- Fiber: 12g

Lunch: Tuna and White Bean Salad

Ingredients

- 1 can white beans (cannellini or navy), drained and rinsed
- 1 can tuna, drained
- 1/4 cup diced red onion
- 1/4 cup diced celery
- 2 tablespoons chopped fresh parsley
- 1 tablespoon lemon juice
- 2 tablespoons olive oil
- Salt and pepper to taste

Instructions

- In a large bowl, combine white beans, tuna, diced red onion, diced celery, and chopped fresh parsley.
- Sprinkle olive oil and lemon juice over the salad. Season with salt and pepper.
- Toss gently to combine.

Nutritional Information (approximate per serving)

- Calories: 300
- Protein: 25g
- Carbohydrates: 25g
- Fat: 12g
- Fiber: 8g

Snack: Greek Yogurt with Mixed Nuts

Ingredients

- 1/2 cup Greek yogurt
- 1/4 cup mixed nuts (almonds, walnuts, cashews)

Instructions

1. Serve Greek yogurt with mixed nuts on top.

Nutritional Information (approximate per serving)

- Calories: 250
- Protein: 18g
- Carbohydrates: 10g
- Fat: 15g
- Fiber: 3g

Dinner: Grilled Salmon with Asparagus

Ingredients

- 6 oz salmon fillet
- 1 bunch asparagus, trimmed
- 1 tablespoon olive oil
- Salt and pepper to taste

Instructions

1. Preheat grill to medium-high heat.
2. Rub asparagus spears and salmon fillet with olive oil. Season with salt and pepper.
3. Grill salmon for about 4-5 minutes on each side until cooked through.
4. Grill asparagus for about 2-3 minutes on each side until tender but still

crisp.

5. Serve grilled salmon with grilled asparagus.

Nutritional Information (approximate per serving)

- Calories: 350
- Protein: 30g
- Carbohydrates: 8g
- Fat: 20g
- Fiber: 4g

Day 5

Breakfast: Avocado and Egg Toast

Ingredients

- 1 slice whole grain bread
- 1/2 avocado
- 1 egg
- Salt and pepper to taste

Instructions

1. Toast the whole grain bread to your desired level of crispiness.
2. While the bread is toasting, slice the avocado and mash it with a fork.
3. Cook the egg according to your preference (fried, scrambled, or poached).
4. Spread the mashed avocado on the toasted bread.
5. Top with the cooked egg and season with salt and pepper.

Nutritional Information (approximate per serving)

- Calories: 300
- Protein: 13g
- Carbohydrates: 20g
- Fat: 20g
- Fiber: 8g

Lunch: Mediterranean Chickpea Wrap

Ingredients

- 1 whole wheat tortilla
- 1/2 cup cooked chickpeas
- 1/4 cup diced cucumber
- 1/4 cup diced tomato
- 2 tablespoons diced red onion
- 2 tablespoons crumbled feta cheese
- 1 tablespoon chopped fresh parsley
- 1 tablespoon hummus

Instructions

1. Warm the whole wheat tortilla slightly.
2. Spread hummus evenly over the tortilla.
3. In the center of the tortilla, layer cooked chickpeas, diced cucumber, diced tomato, diced red onion, crumbled feta cheese, and chopped fresh parsley.
4. Roll the tortilla tightly into a wrap.
5. Cut the wrap in half diagonally before serving.

Nutritional Information (approximate per serving)

- Calories: 350
- Protein: 15g

- Carbohydrates: 45g
- Fat: 12g
- Fiber: 10g

Snack: Apple Slices with Peanut Butter

Ingredients

- 1 apple, sliced
- 2 tablespoons peanut butter

Instructions

1. Slice the apple into wedges.
2. Serve with peanut butter for dipping.

Nutritional Information (approximate per serving)

- Calories: 250
- Protein: 6g
- Carbohydrates: 30g
- Fat: 14g
- Fiber: 7g

Dinner: Baked Cod with Lemon Garlic Butter Sauce

Ingredients

- 6 oz cod fillet
- 1 tablespoon olive oil
- 1 clove garlic, minced
- Zest and juice of 1 lemon
- 2 tablespoons unsalted butter

- Salt and pepper to taste

Instructions

- Preheat oven to 375°F (190°C). Place cod fillet on a baking sheet lined with parchment paper.
- In a saucepan, heat olive oil over medium heat. Add minced garlic and cook until fragrant.
- Add lemon zest, lemon juice, and unsalted butter to the saucepan. Cook until the butter melts and the sauce is well combined.
- Pour the lemon garlic butter sauce over the cod fillet.
- Bake for about 15-20 minutes until the cod is cooked through and flakes easily with a fork.

Nutritional Information (approximate per serving)

- Calories: 300
- Protein: 30g
- Carbohydrates: 2g
- Fat: 20g
- Fiber: 0g

Day 6

Breakfast: Spinach and Tomato Frittata

Ingredients

- 4 large eggs
- 1 cup spinach leaves
- 1/2 cup cherry tomatoes, halved
- 1/4 cup diced onion
- 2 tablespoons grated Parmesan cheese

- Salt and pepper to taste

Instructions

1. Preheat oven to 350°F (175°C).
2. In a bowl, whisk together eggs, pepper and salt.
3. Heat an oven-safe skillet over medium heat. Add diced onion and cook until translucent.
4. Add spinach leaves to the skillet and cook until it sagged.
5. Pour the whisked eggs over the vegetables in the skillet. Sprinkle halved cherry tomatoes and grated Parmesan cheese on top.
6. Cook on the stovetop for 2-3 minutes until the edges start to set.
7. Transfer the skillet to the preheated oven and bake for 10-12 minutes until the frittata is set and golden brown on top.
8. Slice and serve.

Nutritional Information (approximate per serving)

- Calories: 250
- Protein: 18g
- Carbohydrates: 6g
- Fat: 16g
- Fiber: 2g

Lunch: Greek Chicken Salad

Ingredients

- 4 oz grilled chicken breast, sliced
- Mixed salad greens
- 1/4 cup sliced cucumber
- 1/4 cup sliced cherry tomatoes
- 2 tablespoons sliced red onion

- 2 tablespoons crumbled feta cheese
- Greek vinaigrette dressing

Instructions

1. Arrange mixed salad greens on a plate.
2. Top with sliced grilled chicken breast, sliced cucumber, sliced cherry tomatoes, sliced red onion, and crumbled feta cheese.
3. Drizzle with Greek vinaigrette dressing.

Nutritional Information (approximate per serving)

- Calories: 300
- Protein: 30g
- Carbohydrates: 10g
- Fat: 15g
- Fiber: 4g

Snack: Greek Yogurt with Berries

Ingredients

- 1/2 cup Greek yogurt
- 1/4 cup mixed berries (strawberries, blueberries, raspberries)

Instructions

1. Serve Greek yogurt topped with mixed berries.

Nutritional Information (approximate per serving)

- Calories: 150
- Protein: 12g
- Carbohydrates: 15g
- Fat: 5g

- Fiber: 3g

Dinner: Mediterranean Grilled Vegetable Platter

Ingredients

- Assorted vegetables (bell peppers, zucchini, eggplant, cherry tomatoes), sliced
- 2 tablespoons olive oil
- 1 tablespoon balsamic vinegar
- 2 cloves garlic, minced
- Salt and pepper to taste

Instructions

1. Preheat grill to medium-high heat.
2. In a bowl, toss sliced vegetables with olive oil, balsamic vinegar, minced garlic, salt, and pepper.
3. Grill vegetables for about 3-4 minutes on each side until tender and charred.
4. Arrange grilled vegetables on a platter and serve.

Nutritional Information (approximate per serving)

- Calories: 250
- Protein: 5g
- Carbohydrates: 20g
- Fat: 18g
- Fiber: 8g

Day 7

Breakfast: Greek Yogurt Parfait

Ingredients

- 1/2 cup Greek yogurt
- 1/4 cup granola
- 1/4 cup mixed berries (strawberries, blueberries, raspberries)
- 1 tablespoon honey (optional)

Instructions

1. In a bowl or glass layer Greek yogurt, mixed berries and granola.
2. Repeat the layers until all ingredients are used.
3. Drizzle with honey if desired.

Nutritional Information (approximate per serving)

- Calories: 300
- Protein: 15g
- Carbohydrates: 40g
- Fat: 10g
- Fiber: 6g

Lunch: Quinoa and Vegetable Stuffed Bell Peppers

Ingredients

- 2 large bell peppers, halved and seeded
- 1 cup cooked quinoa
- 1/2 cup black beans, drained and rinsed
- 1/2 cup corn kernels
- 1/4 cup diced tomatoes
- 1/4 cup diced red onion

- 1/4 cup chopped fresh cilantro
- 1 teaspoon ground cumin
- 1/2 teaspoon chili powder
- Salt and pepper to taste

Instructions

1. Preheat oven to 375°F (190°C). Place bell pepper halves in a baking dish.
2. In a large bowl, combine cooked quinoa, black beans, corn kernels, diced tomatoes, diced red onion, chopped fresh cilantro, ground cumin, chili powder, salt, and pepper.
3. Spoon the quinoa mixture into each bell pepper half.
4. Bake for about 25-30 minutes until the bell peppers are tender.

Nutritional Information (approximate per serving)

- Calories: 350
- Protein: 15g
- Carbohydrates: 60g
- Fat: 5g
- Fiber: 12g

Snack: Carrot Sticks with Hummus

Ingredients

- 1 carrot, cut into sticks
- 1/4 cup hummus

Instructions

Serve carrot sticks with hummus for dipping.
Nutritional Information (approximate per serving)

- Calories: 100
- Protein: 3g
- Carbohydrates: 15g
- Fat: 4g
- Fiber: 6g

Dinner: Lemon Herb Grilled Shrimp Skewers

Ingredients

- 8 oz shrimp, peeled and deveined
- 1 tablespoon olive oil
- Zest and juice of 1 lemon
- 2 cloves garlic, minced
- 1 tablespoon chopped fresh parsley
- 1 tablespoon chopped fresh dill
- Salt and pepper to taste

Instructions

1. In a bowl, whisk together olive oil, lemon zest, lemon juice, minced garlic, chopped fresh parsley, chopped fresh dill, salt, and pepper.
2. Thread shrimp onto skewers.
3. Brush the marinade over the shrimp skewers.
4. Preheat grill to medium-high heat. Grill shrimp skewers for about 2-3 minutes on each side until pink and opaque.
5. Serve hot.

Nutritional Information (approximate per serving)

- Calories: 250
- Protein: 25g
- Carbohydrates: 3g

- Fat: 15g
- Fiber: 0g

Day 1 (Week 3)

Breakfast: Mediterranean Omelette

Ingredients

- 2 large eggs
- 1/4 cup diced tomatoes
- 1/4 cup chopped spinach
- 2 tablespoons diced red onion
- 2 tablespoons crumbled feta cheese
- 1 tablespoon chopped fresh parsley
- Salt and pepper to taste

Instructions

1. In a bowl, whisk together eggs, pepper and salt.
2. Heat a non-stick skillet over medium heat. Pour the whisked eggs into the skillet.
3. Cook until the edges start to set, then sprinkle diced tomatoes, chopped spinach, diced red onion, crumbled feta cheese, and chopped fresh parsley over one half of the omelette.
4. Fold the other half of the omelette over the filling.
5. Cook for another 1-2 minutes until the filling is heated through and the eggs are cooked to your desired doneness.
6. Slide the omelette onto a plate and serve.

Nutritional Information (approximate per serving)

- Calories: 300
- Protein: 18g
- Carbohydrates: 8g
- Fat: 20g
- Fiber: 2g

Lunch: Greek Chicken Pita Wrap

Ingredients

- 4 oz grilled chicken breast, sliced
- 1 whole wheat pita bread
- 2 tablespoons tzatziki sauce
- 1/4 cup sliced cucumber
- 1/4 cup sliced tomatoes
- 2 tablespoons sliced red onion
- 1 tablespoon chopped fresh parsley

Instructions

1. Warm the whole wheat pita bread slightly.
2. Spread tzatziki sauce evenly inside the pita.
3. Fill the pita with sliced grilled chicken breast, sliced cucumber, sliced tomatoes, sliced red onion, and chopped fresh parsley.
4. Serve immediately.

Nutritional Information (approximate per serving)

- Calories: 350
- Protein: 30g
- Carbohydrates: 30g
- Fat: 12g
- Fiber: 6g

Snack: Greek Yogurt with Honey and Pistachios

Ingredients

- 1/2 cup Greek yogurt
- 1 tablespoon honey
- 2 tablespoons chopped pistachios

Instructions

1. In a bowl, combine Greek yogurt and honey.
2. Top with chopped pistachios.

Nutritional Information (approximate per serving)

- Calories: 250
- Protein: 15g
- Carbohydrates: 20g
- Fat: 12g
- Fiber: 2g

Dinner: Grilled Vegetable and Halloumi Skewers

Ingredients

- Assorted vegetables (bell peppers, zucchini, cherry tomatoes, mush-rooms), cut into chunks
- 4 oz halloumi cheese, cut into cubes
- 2 tablespoons olive oil
- 1 tablespoon balsamic vinegar
- Salt and pepper to taste

Instructions

1. Preheat grill to medium-high heat.
2. Thread alternating pieces of vegetables and halloumi cheese onto skewers.
3. In a bowl, whisk together olive oil, balsamic vinegar, salt, and pepper.
4. Brush the marinade over the skewers.
5. Grill skewers for about 3-4 minutes on each side until the vegetables are tender and the halloumi cheese is lightly charred.
6. Serve hot.

Nutritional Information (approximate per serving)

- Calories: 300
- Protein: 15g
- Carbohydrates: 15g
- Fat: 20g
- Fiber: 5g

Day 2

Breakfast: Berry and Almond Butter Smoothie Bowl

Ingredients

- 1/2 cup mixed berries (strawberries, blueberries, raspberries)
- 1/2 banana
- 1/2 cup any milk of your choice)
- 2 tablespoons almond butter
- 1 tablespoon honey (optional)
- Toppings: sliced almonds, shredded coconut, chia seeds, additional berries

Instructions

1. In a blender, combine mixed berries, banana, almond milk, almond butter, and honey.
2. Blend until smooth.
3. Pour the smoothie into a bowl.
4. Top with sliced almonds, shredded coconut, chia seeds, and additional berries.

Nutritional Information (approximate per serving)

- Calories: 350
- Protein: 8g
- Carbohydrates: 40g
- Fat: 20g
- Fiber: 8g

Lunch: Mediterranean Chickpea Salad

Ingredients

- 1 can chickpeas, drained and rinsed
- 1/2 cucumber, diced
- 1/2 cup cherry tomatoes, halved
- 1/4 cup diced red onion
- 1/4 cup chopped fresh parsley
- 2 tablespoons crumbled feta cheese
- 2 tablespoons olive oil
- 1 tablespoon lemon juice
- 1 teaspoon dried oregano
- Salt and pepper to taste

Instructions

1. In a large bowl, combine chickpeas, diced cucumber, cherry tomatoes,

diced red onion, chopped fresh parsley, and crumbled feta cheese.

2. In a bowl, whisk together olive oil, dried oregano, lemon juice, pepper and salt to make the dressing.

3. Pour the dressing over the salad and toss to combine.

4. Serve chilled or at room temperature.

Nutritional Information (approximate per serving)

- Calories: 300
- Protein: 10g
- Carbohydrates: 30g
- Fat: 15g
- Fiber: 8g

Snack: Sliced Cucumber with Hummus

Ingredients

- 1 cucumber, sliced
- 1/4 cup hummus

Instructions

1. Serve sliced cucumber with hummus for dipping.

Nutritional Information (approximate per serving)

- Calories: 100
- Protein: 4g
- Carbohydrates: 10g
- Fat: 6g
- Fiber: 4g

Dinner: Grilled Swordfish with Lemon Herb Marinade

Ingredients

- 6 oz swordfish steak
- 2 tablespoons olive oil
- Zest and juice of 1 lemon
- 2 cloves garlic, minced
- 1 tablespoon chopped fresh parsley
- 1 tablespoon chopped fresh dill
- Salt and pepper to taste

Instructions

1. In a bowl, whisk together olive oil, lemon zest, lemon juice, minced garlic, chopped fresh parsley, chopped fresh dill, salt, and pepper to make the marinade.
2. Place swordfish steak in a shallow dish and pour the marinade over it. Make sure the fish is well coated. Marinate in the refrigerator for at least 30 minutes.
3. Preheat grill to medium-high heat. Remove swordfish from the marinade and discard excess marinade.
4. Grill swordfish for about 3-4 minutes on each side until cooked through and grill marks appear.
5. Serve hot.

Nutritional Information (approximate per serving)

- Calories: 350
- Protein: 30g
- Carbohydrates: 2g
- Fat: 25g
- Fiber: 0g

Day 3

Breakfast: Mediterranean Breakfast Bowl

Ingredients

- 1/2 cup cooked quinoa
- 1/4 cup diced cucumber
- 1/4 cup halved cherry tomatoes
- 2 tablespoons diced red onion
- 2 tablespoons crumbled feta cheese
- 1 tablespoon chopped fresh parsley
- 1 tablespoon olive oil
- 1 tablespoon lemon juice
- Salt and pepper to taste

Instructions

1. In a bowl, combine cooked quinoa, diced cucumber, halved cherry tomatoes, diced red onion, crumbled feta cheese, and chopped fresh parsley.
2. Drizzle olive oil and lemon juice over the ingredients.
3. Season with salt and pepper to taste.
4. Toss gently to combine.

Nutritional Information (approximate per serving)

- Calories: 300
- Protein: 8g
- Carbohydrates: 30g
- Fat: 15g
- Fiber: 5g

Lunch: Greek Salad with Grilled Chicken

Ingredients

- Mixed salad greens
- 4 oz grilled chicken breast, sliced
- 1/4 cup sliced cucumber
- 1/4 cup sliced cherry tomatoes
- 2 tablespoons sliced red onion
- 2 tablespoons crumbled feta cheese
- Greek vinaigrette dressing

Instructions

1. Arrange mixed salad greens on a plate.
2. Top with sliced grilled chicken breast, sliced cucumber, sliced cherry tomatoes, sliced red onion, and crumbled feta cheese.
3. Drizzle with Greek vinaigrette dressing.

Nutritional Information (approximate per serving)

- Calories: 350
- Protein: 30g
- Carbohydrates: 10g
- Fat: 20g
- Fiber: 4g

Snack: Greek Yogurt with Berries and Walnuts

Ingredients

- 1/2 cup Greek yogurt
- 1/4 cup mixed berries (strawberries, blueberries, raspberries)

- 2 tablespoons chopped walnuts

Instructions

1. Serve Greek yogurt topped with mixed berries and chopped walnuts.

Nutritional Information (approximate per serving)

- Calories: 250
- Protein: 15g
- Carbohydrates: 15g
- Fat: 15g
- Fiber: 3g

Dinner: Lemon Garlic Shrimp Pasta

Ingredients

- 6 oz whole wheat pasta
- 6 oz shrimp, peeled and deveined
- 2 tablespoons olive oil
- 2 cloves garlic, minced
- Zest and juice of 1 lemon
- Salt and pepper to taste
- Fresh parsley, chopped (for garnish)

Instructions

1. Cook pasta according to package instructions. Drain and set aside.
2. In skillet, heat olive oil over medium heat. Add minced garlic and cook until fragrant.
3. Add shrimp to the skillet and cook until pink and opaque.
4. Stir in lemon zest and juice. Season with salt and pepper.

5. Add cooked pasta to the skillet and toss to coat with the lemon garlic sauce.
6. Serve hot, garnished with chopped fresh parsley.

Nutritional Information (approximate per serving)

- Calories: 400
- Protein: 25g
- Carbohydrates: 45g
- Fat: 15g
- Fiber: 8g

Day 4

Breakfast: Mediterranean Veggie Omelette

Ingredients

- 2 large eggs
- 1/4 cup diced bell peppers (any color)
- 1/4 cup diced tomatoes
- 2 tablespoons diced red onion
- 2 tablespoons chopped spinach
- 2 tablespoons crumbled feta cheese
- Salt and pepper to taste

Instructions

1. In a bowl, whisk together eggs, pepper and salt.
2. Heat a non-stick skillet over medium heat and coat it lightly with cooking spray.
3. Pour the whisked eggs into the skillet.
4. As the eggs begin to set, sprinkle diced bell peppers, diced tomatoes,

diced red onion, chopped spinach, and crumbled feta cheese evenly over one half of the omelette.

5. Cook until the bottom is set and the cheese begins to melt.
6. Fold the other half of the omelette over the filling.
7. Cook for another minute or until the omelette is cooked through.
8. Slide onto a plate and serve.

Nutritional Information (approximate per serving)

- Calories: 250
- Protein: 18g
- Carbohydrates: 8g
- Fat: 15g
- Fiber: 2g

Lunch: Greek-style Quinoa Salad

Ingredients

- 1 cup cooked quinoa
- 1/4 cup diced cucumber
- 1/4 cup diced tomatoes
- 2 tablespoons diced red onion
- 2 tablespoons chopped Kalamata olives
- 2 tablespoons crumbled feta cheese
- 1 tablespoon chopped fresh parsley
- 1 tablespoon olive oil
- 1 tablespoon lemon juice
- Salt and pepper to taste

Instructions

1. In a large bowl, combine cooked quinoa, diced cucumber, diced

tomatoes, diced red onion, chopped Kalamata olives, crumbled feta cheese, and chopped fresh parsley.

2. In a bowl, whisk together olive oil, lemon juice, pepper and salt to make the dressing.

3. Pour the dressing over the salad and toss to combine.

4. Serve chilled or at room temperature.

Nutritional Information (approximate per serving)

- Calories: 300
- Protein: 10g
- Carbohydrates: 35g
- Fat: 15g
- Fiber: 6g

Snack: Greek Yogurt with Honey and Almonds

Ingredients

- 1/2 cup Greek yogurt
- 1 tablespoon honey
- 2 tablespoons chopped almonds

Instructions

1. In a bowl, combine Greek yogurt and honey.
2. Top with chopped almonds.

Nutritional Information (approximate per serving)

- Calories: 250
- Protein: 15g
- Carbohydrates: 20g

- Fat: 12g
- Fiber: 2g

Dinner: Baked Mediterranean Cod

Ingredients

- 6 oz cod fillet
- 1/4 cup diced tomatoes
- 1/4 cup chopped Kalamata olives
- 2 tablespoons diced red onion
- 1 tablespoon capers
- 1 tablespoon olive oil
- 1 tablespoon lemon juice
- 1 teaspoon dried oregano
- Salt and pepper to taste

Instructions

- Preheat oven to 375°F (190°C). Place cod fillet in a baking dish.
- In a bowl, mix together diced tomatoes, chopped Kalamata olives, diced red onion, capers, olive oil, lemon juice, dried oregano, salt, and pepper.
- Spoon the mixture over the cod fillet.
- Bake for about 15-20 minutes until the fish is cooked through and flakes easily with a fork.
- Serve hot.

Nutritional Information (approximate per serving)

- Calories: 300
- Protein: 30g
- Carbohydrates: 8g
- Fat: 15g

- Fiber: 2g

Day 5

Breakfast: Mediterranean Breakfast Wrap

Ingredients

- 1 whole wheat tortilla
- 2 eggs, scrambled
- 1/4 cup diced tomatoes
- 2 tablespoons chopped spinach
- 2 tablespoons crumbled feta cheese
- Salt and pepper to taste

Instructions

1. Heat the whole wheat tortilla in a skillet or microwave until warm.
2. In the center of the tortilla, layer scrambled eggs, diced tomatoes, chopped spinach, and crumbled feta cheese.
3. Season with salt and pepper.
4. Fold in the sides of the tortilla and roll up tightly to form a wrap.
5. Serve immediately.

Nutritional Information (approximate per serving)

- Calories: 350
- Protein: 20g
- Carbohydrates: 25g
- Fat: 18g
- Fiber: 5g

Lunch: Greek-style Lentil Salad

Ingredients

1. 1 cup cooked lentils
2. 1/4 cup diced cucumber
3. 1/4 cup diced tomatoes
4. 2 tablespoons diced red onion
5. 2 tablespoons chopped Kalamata olives
6. 2 tablespoons crumbled feta cheese
7. 1 tablespoon chopped fresh parsley
8. 1 tablespoon olive oil
9. 1 tablespoon red wine vinegar
10. Salt and pepper to taste

Instructions

1. In a large bowl, combine cooked lentils, diced cucumber, diced tomatoes, diced red onion, chopped Kalamata olives, crumbled feta cheese, and chopped fresh parsley.
2. In a bowl, whisk together olive oil, red wine vinegar, pepper and salt to make the dressing.
3. Pour the dressing over the salad and toss to combine.
4. Serve chilled or at room temperature.

Nutritional Information (approximate per serving)

- Calories: 300
- Protein: 15g
- Carbohydrates: 35g
- Fat: 12g
- Fiber: 10g

Snack: Greek Yogurt with Granola and Honey

Ingredients

- 1/2 cup Greek yogurt
- 1/4 cup granola
- 1 tablespoon honey

Instructions

1. In a bowl, layer Greek yogurt, granola, and drizzle with honey.

Nutritional Information (approximate per serving)

- Calories: 250
- Protein: 12g
- Carbohydrates: 30g
- Fat: 10g
- Fiber: 4g

Dinner: Mediterranean Stuffed Bell Peppers

Ingredients

- 2 large bell peppers, halved and seeded
- 1 cup cooked quinoa
- 1/2 cup diced tomatoes
- 1/2 cup chopped spinach
- 1/4 cup diced red onion
- 1/4 cup crumbled feta cheese
- 2 tablespoons chopped Kalamata olives
- 1 tablespoon olive oil
- 1 tablespoon lemon juice

- 1 teaspoon dried oregano
- Salt and pepper to taste

Instructions

1. Preheat oven to 375°F (190°C). Place bell pepper halves in a baking dish.
2. In a large bowl, combine cooked quinoa, diced tomatoes, chopped spinach, diced red onion, crumbled feta cheese, chopped Kalamata olives, olive oil, lemon juice, dried oregano, salt, and pepper.
3. Spoon the quinoa mixture into each bell pepper half.
4. Cover the baking dish with foil and bake for about 25-30 minutes.
5. Serve hot.

Nutritional Information (approximate per serving)

- Calories: 350
- Protein: 12g
- Carbohydrates: 45g
- Fat: 15g
- Fiber: 8g

Day 6

Breakfast: Greek Yogurt Parfait

Ingredients

- 1/2 cup Greek yogurt
- 1/4 cup granola
- 1/4 cup mixed berries (strawberries, blueberries, raspberries)
- 1 tablespoon honey (optional)

Instructions

1. In a bowl or glass, layer Greek yogurt, mixed berries and granola.
2. Repeat the layers until all ingredients are used.
3. Drizzle with honey if desired.

Nutritional Information (approximate per serving)

- Calories: 300
- Protein: 15g
- Carbohydrates: 40g
- Fat: 10g
- Fiber: 6g

Lunch: Mediterranean Chickpea Wraps

Ingredients

- 1 whole wheat tortilla
- 1/2 cup cooked chickpeas, mashed
- 2 tablespoons diced tomatoes
- 2 tablespoons diced cucumber
- 2 tablespoons diced red onion
- 2 tablespoons chopped fresh parsley
- 1 tablespoon lemon juice
- 1 tablespoon olive oil
- Salt and pepper to taste

Instructions

1. In a bowl, mix together mashed chickpeas, diced tomatoes, diced cucumber, diced red onion, chopped fresh parsley, lemon juice, olive oil, salt, and pepper.
2. Spread the chickpea mixture onto the whole wheat tortilla.
3. Roll up the tortilla tightly to form a wrap.

4. Cut the wrap in half and serve.

Nutritional Information (approximate per serving)

- Calories: 350
- Protein: 12g
- Carbohydrates: 45g
- Fat: 15g
- Fiber: 8g

Snack: Hummus with Veggie Sticks

Ingredients

- 1/4 cup hummus
- Assorted veggie sticks (carrots, cucumber, bell peppers)

Instructions

1. Serve hummus with veggie sticks for dipping.

Nutritional Information (approximate per serving)

- Calories: 150
- Protein: 6g
- Carbohydrates: 15g
- Fat: 8g
- Fiber: 6g

Dinner: Lemon Herb Grilled Chicken

Ingredients

- 6 oz chicken breast

- 1 tablespoon olive oil
- Zest and juice of 1 lemon
- 2 cloves garlic, minced
- 1 tablespoon chopped fresh parsley
- 1 tablespoon chopped fresh thyme
- Salt and pepper to taste

Instructions

1. In a bowl, whisk together olive oil, lemon zest, lemon juice, minced garlic, chopped fresh parsley, chopped fresh thyme, salt, and pepper.
2. Place chicken breast in a shallow dish and pour the marinade over it. Make sure the chicken is well coated. Marinate in the refrigerator for at least 30 minutes.
3. Preheat grill to medium-high heat. Remove chicken from the marinade and discard excess marinade.
4. Grill chicken for about 6-8 minutes on each side until cooked through and no longer pink in the center.
5. Serve hot.

Nutritional Information (approximate per serving)

- Calories: 300
- Protein: 40g
- Carbohydrates: 2g
- Fat: 12g
- Fiber: 0g

Day 7

Breakfast: Greek Yogurt with Berries and Almonds

Ingredients

- 1/2 cup Greek yogurt
- 1/4 cup mixed berries (strawberries, blueberries, raspberries)
- 2 tablespoons sliced almonds
- 1 tablespoon honey (optional)

Instructions

1. In a bowl, layer Greek yogurt and mixed berries.
2. Sprinkle sliced almonds on top.
3. Drizzle with honey if desired.

Nutritional Information (approximate per serving):

- Calories: 250
- Protein: 15g
- Carbohydrates: 20g
- Fat: 12g
- Fiber: 4g

Lunch: Mediterranean Veggie Wrap

Ingredients

- 1 whole wheat tortilla
- 2 tablespoons hummus
- 1/4 cup sliced cucumber
- 1/4 cup sliced bell peppers (any color)
- 1/4 cup sliced tomatoes
- 2 tablespoons crumbled feta cheese
- 1 tablespoon chopped fresh parsley

Instructions

1. Spread hummus evenly onto the whole wheat tortilla.
2. Layer sliced cucumber, sliced bell peppers, sliced tomatoes, crumbled feta cheese, and chopped fresh parsley on top of the hummus.
3. Roll up the tortilla tightly to form a wrap.
4. Cut the wrap in half and serve.

Nutritional Information (approximate per serving)

- Calories: 300
- Protein: 10g
- Carbohydrates: 35g
- Fat: 15g
- Fiber: 8g

Snack: Greek Yogurt with Granola and Fruit

Ingredients

- 1/2 cup Greek yogurt
- 1/4 cup granola
- 1/4 cup diced fresh fruit (such as banana, apple, or kiwi)

Instructions

1. In a bowl, layer Greek yogurt, granola, and diced fresh fruit.
Nutritional Information (approximate per serving):

- Calories: 300
- Protein: 15g
- Carbohydrates: 40g
- Fat: 10g
- Fiber: 6g

Dinner: Baked Salmon with Lemon and Dill

Ingredients

- 6 oz salmon fillet
- 1 tablespoon olive oil
- Zest and juice of 1 lemon
- 1 tablespoon chopped fresh dill
- Salt and pepper to taste

Instructions

1. Preheat oven to 375°F (190°C). Place salmon fillet on a baking sheet lined with parchment paper.
2. In a bowl, whisk together olive oil, lemon zest, lemon juice, chopped fresh dill, salt, and pepper.
3. Pour the marinade over the salmon fillet, spreading it evenly.
4. Bake for about 12-15 minutes until the salmon is cooked through and flakes easily with a fork.
5. Serve hot.

Nutritional Information (approximate per serving)

- Calories: 350
- Protein: 30g
- Carbohydrates: 2g
- Fat: 25g
- Fiber: 0g

Vegetarian and Vegan Options

If you are following a vegetarian or vegan lifestyle, the Atlantic diet offers plenty of delicious and nutritious options. Here are some vegetarian and vegan options that align with the principles of the Atlantic diet:

1. Plant-Based Proteins

- Legumes: Beans, lentils, and chickpeas are excellent sources of plant-based protein and can be used in a variety of dishes such as salads, soups, stews, and veggie burgers.
- Tofu and Tempeh: These soy-based products are versatile protein sources that can be marinated, grilled, sautéed, or added to stir-fries and salads.
- Seitan: Made from wheat gluten, seitan is a high-protein meat substitute that can be used in place of chicken or beef in dishes like stir-fries, sandwiches, and tacos.
- Edamame: These young soybeans are rich in protein and can be enjoyed as a snack, added to salads, or used in stir-fries and grain bowls.

2. Whole Grains

- Quinoa: A complete protein, quinoa is a nutritious grain that can be used as a base for salads, pilafs, and breakfast bowls.
- Brown Rice: High in fiber and vitamins, brown rice is a versatile grain that pairs well with vegetables, legumes, and tofu.
- Bulgur: A quick-cooking grain, bulgur is often used in Mediterranean salads like tabbouleh and can also be added to soups and pilafs.

3. Healthy Fats

- Avocado: Rich in heart-healthy monounsaturated fats, avocado is a versatile ingredient that can be used in salads, sandwiches, wraps, and smoothies.

- Nuts and Seeds: Almonds, walnuts, chia seeds, flaxseeds, and hemp seeds are excellent sources of healthy fats, protein, and fiber. Enjoy them as a snack, sprinkle them on salads and yogurt, or use them in baking and cooking.

4. Dairy Alternatives

- Plant-Based Milk: Opt for unsweetened almond milk, coconut milk, or oat milk as dairy alternatives in recipes, smoothies, and cereal.
- Vegan Cheese: Look for dairy-free cheese alternatives made from nuts, soy, or coconut to use in recipes like pizzas, pasta dishes, and sandwiches.

5. Fruits and Vegetables

- Load up on a variety of fresh fruits and vegetables to ensure a diverse and balanced diet. Incorporate seasonal produce into your meals for maximum flavor and nutritional benefits.
- Leafy greens like spinach, kale, and Swiss chard are rich in vitamins, minerals, and antioxidants and can be enjoyed raw in salads or cooked in soups, stews, and stir-fries.

6. Eggs and Dairy Substitutes

- Vegetarians may choose to include eggs and dairy products like Greek yogurt and feta cheese in their diet. For vegans, there are plenty of plant-based alternatives available, such as tofu scrambles, coconut yogurt, and dairy-free cheese.

7. Ethnic Cuisine Inspiration

- Explore Mediterranean-inspired vegetarian and vegan dishes like falafel, hummus, tabbouleh, stuffed grape leaves, ratatouille, and vegetable paella for flavorful and satisfying meals.

5

Chapter 4: Tips for Healthy Cooking

1. Use Healthy Cooking Methods

Opt for healthy cooking methods that preserve the nutritional integrity of foods while minimizing added fats and calories. Examples include:

- Steaming: Steaming vegetables helps retain their vitamins, minerals, and natural flavors without added fat.
- Grilling: Grilling meats, seafood, and vegetables adds flavor without the need for excessive oil or butter.
- Baking or Roasting: Baking or roasting foods in the oven with minimal oil allows them to caramelize and develop rich flavors.
- Sautéing: Sauté vegetables, proteins, and grains in a small amount of olive oil or vegetable broth for added flavor and moisture.
- Poaching: Poaching fish, chicken, or eggs in simmering liquid helps retain moisture and yields tender, flavorful results.

2. Limit Added Fats and Sugars

- Be mindful of the amount of added fats and sugars used in cooking. Instead of frying foods or drenching them in heavy sauces, opt for lighter alternatives such as herbs, spices, citrus juices, and vinegar for flavor.
- Use healthier fats like extra-virgin olive oil, avocado oil, or coconut oil in moderation, and avoid highly processed oils and trans fats.

3. Load Up on Fruits and Vegetables

- Incorporate plenty of fruits and vegetables into your meals to boost fiber, vitamins, minerals, and antioxidants.Experiment with different cooking methods for vegetables, such as roasting, grilling, steaming, or stir-frying, to enhance their flavors and textures.

4. Choose Lean Proteins

- Select lean protein sources such as poultry, fish, legumes, tofu, and tempeh to reduce saturated fat intake. Remove skin from poultry and trim visible fat from meats before cooking.
- Incorporate plant-based proteins like beans, lentils, and quinoa into your meals to increase fiber and reduce the consumption of animal products.

5. Include Whole Grains

- Choose whole grains such as brown rice, quinoa, barley, farro, and whole wheat pasta over refined grains for added fiber, vitamins, and minerals.
- Experiment with different whole grains in your recipes to add variety and texture to your meals.

6. Practice Portion Control

- Be mindful of portion sizes to avoid overeating and unnecessary calorie consumption. Use smaller plates to help control portion sizes and prevent overeating.
- Pay attention to hunger and fullness cues and stop eating when you feel satisfied, rather than continuing to eat until you're uncomfortably full.

7. Minimize Sodium Intake

- Limit the amount of added salt in your cooking and opt for herbs, spices, citrus zest, and vinegar to enhance flavor instead.
- Choose low-sodium or no-salt-added versions of canned and packaged foods, and rinse canned beans and vegetables before using them to reduce sodium content.

8. Stay Hydrated

- Drink plenty of water throughout the day to stay hydrated and support your overall health. Limit sugary beverages like soda, fruit juices, and energy drinks, and opt for water, herbal tea, or infused water instead.

9. Plan Ahead and Prepare Meals at Home

- Plan your meals ahead of time and prepare homemade meals as often as possible. Cooking at home allows you to have full control over the ingredients used and enables you to make healthier choices.

10. Enjoy the Process

Cooking can be a fun and enjoyable activity, so embrace the process and experiment with new ingredients, flavors, and recipes. Get creative in the kitchen and involve friends or family members in meal preparation for added enjoyment.

6

Chapter 5: Long-Term Sustainability and Health Maintenance

Building Healthy Habits

Building healthy habits is a gradual process that requires realistic goal-setting, consistency, and patience. Start by setting achievable goals and creating a clear plan for how you'll reach them. Begin with small, manageable changes and track your progress along the way. Stay flexible and adapt your plan as needed, and seek support from friends, family, or communities with similar goals. Focus on behavior change rather than fixating on outcomes, and remember that building healthy habits takes time. By incorporating these strategies into your daily life and staying committed to your journey, you can create lasting habits that support your overall health and well-being.

Preventing Plateaus

Preventing plateaus in your health and wellness journey is crucial for maintaining progress and momentum. Regularly assess your progress, mix up your routine with variety in exercise and diet, and progressively overload your workouts. Incorporate rest and recovery, make nutritional adjustments, and manage stress effectively. Seek professional guidance if needed. By implementing these strategies, you can overcome plateaus and continue moving forward toward your goals with resilience and adaptability.

7

Chapter 6: Comprehensive Atlantic Diet Food List

1. Seafood

- Salmon
- Cod
- Tuna
- Mackerel
- Sardines
- Shrimp
- Crab
- Lobster
- Clams
- Oysters
- Scallops
- Anchovies
- Haddock
- Trout
- Herring
- Swordfish

- Sea bass
- Hake

2. Vegetables

- Spinach
- Kale
- Swiss chard
- Broccoli
- Cauliflower
- Brussels sprouts
- Tomatoes
- Bell peppers (red, green, yellow)
- Cucumbers
- Zucchini
- Eggplant
- Asparagus
- Artichokes
- Green beans
- Peas
- Carrots
- Beets
- Radishes
- Lettuce (various types)

3. Fruits

- Berries (strawberries, blueberries, raspberries, blackberries)
- Citrus fruits (oranges, lemons, limes)
- Apples
- Bananas
- Pineapple
- Mangoes

- Kiwi
- Papaya
- Avocado
- Melons (watermelon, cantaloupe, honeydew)
- Grapes
- Pears
- Peaches
- Plums

4. Whole Grains

- Quinoa
- Brown rice
- Farro
- Barley
- Bulgur
- Oats
- Whole wheat pasta
- Buckwheat
- Millet
- Cornmeal
- Whole grain bread
- Rye

5. Legumes

- Chickpeas
- Lentils
- Black beans
- Kidney beans
- Navy beans
- Cannellini beans

- Pinto beans
- Split peas
- Edamame
- Fava beans

6. Nuts and Seeds

- Almonds
- Walnuts
- Pecans
- Cashews
- Pistachios
- Hazelnuts
- Macadamia nuts
- Brazil nuts
- Sunflower seeds
- Pumpkin seeds
- Flaxseeds
- Chia seeds
- Sesame seeds

7. Dairy and Dairy Alternatives

- Greek yogurt
- Cottage cheese
- Feta cheese
- Goat cheese
- Parmesan cheese
- Milk (cow's milk, almond milk, soy milk)
- Yogurt (plain, unsweetened)
- Kefir

8. Herbs and Spices

- Basil
- Parsley
- Cilantro
- Dill
- Mint
- Rosemary
- Thyme
- Oregano
- Sage
- Bay leaves
- Garlic
- Ginger
- Turmeric
- Cumin
- Paprika
- Chili powder
- Black pepper
- Sea salt

9. Healthy Fats and Oils

- Olive oil
- Avocado oil
- Coconut oil
- Flaxseed oil
- Walnut oil

10. Beverages

- Water
- Herbal tea
- Green tea
- Coffee (in moderation)
- Red wine (in moderation, if desired)

11. Other

- Honey
- Vinegar (balsamic, red wine, apple cider)
- Olives (green, black)
- Dark chocolate (70% cocoa or higher)

8

CONCLUSION

"The Atlantic Diet Meal Plan" isn't just a collection of recipes—it's a culinary journey that celebrates the vibrant flavors, nourishing ingredients, and timeless traditions of the Mediterranean. As we bid farewell to these pages, may the dishes you've prepared fill your days with joy, your tables with laughter, and your hearts with the warmth of shared meals and cherished memories.

With each bite, may you be reminded of the simple pleasures that come from savoring good food and good company. And as you continue your culinary adventures beyond these recipes, may you carry the spirit of the Atlantic diet with you—a spirit of health, happiness, and a deep appreciation for the beauty of the world around us.

So here's to many more delicious meals, to new culinary discoveries, and to the endless joy of cooking with love. Thank you for joining us on this flavorful journey, and may your kitchen always be filled with the aromas of fresh herbs, ripe tomatoes, and the salty sea breeze. Buon appetito!

Monday	Breakfast	Lunch	Dinner

Tuesday	Breakfast	Lunch	Dinner

Wednesday	Breakfast	Lunch	Dinner

Thursday	Breakfast	Lunch	Dinner

Friday	Breakfast	Lunch	Dinner

Saturday	Breakfast	Lunch	Dinner

Sunday	Breakfast	Lunch	Dinner

Monday

	Breakfast	Lunch	Dinner

Tuesday

	Breakfast	Lunch	Dinner

Wednesday

	Breakfast	Lunch	Dinner

Thursday

	Breakfast	Lunch	Dinner

Friday

	Breakfast	Lunch	Dinner

Saturday

	Breakfast	Lunch	Dinner

Sunday

	Breakfast	Lunch	Dinner